THE PAIN OF CANCER

Understanding and managing cancer
pain with excellence and empathy

Dr Marie Joseph MBBS FRCP

Consultant Lead for Palliative Medicine
(with expertise in complex cancer pain management)
East and North Hertfordshire NHS Trust,
Lister Hospital, Stevenage, Mount Vernon Cancer
Centre, Northwood, and
RCP Educator.

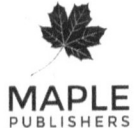

The Pain of Cancer

Author: Dr Marie Joseph

Copyright © Dr Marie Joseph (2022)

The right of Dr Marie Joseph to be identified as author of this work has been asserted by the author in accordance with section 77 and 78 of the Copyright, Designs and Patents Act 1988.

First Published in 2022

ISBN 978-1-915492-51-7 (Paperback)
978-1-915492-61-6 (eBook)

Book cover design and Book layout by:

    White Magic Studios
    www.whitemagicstudios.co.uk

Published by:

    Maple Publishers
    1 Brunel Way,
    Slough,
    SL1 1FQ, UK
    www.maplepublishers.com

A CIP catalogue record for this title is available from the British Library.

All rights reserved. No part of this book may be reproduced or translated by any form or by any means, electronic or mechanical, including photocopying, recording or by any information storage and retrieval system without written permission from the author.

The views expressed in this work are solely those of the author and do not necessarily reflect the views of the publisher, and the publisher hereby disclaims any responsibility for them.

**To watch another's pain is harder than
to endure one's own.**

― *Dr Marie Joseph*

Dedication

In loving memory of my dear parents, Isaac and Mary Casinader for their life-long love, support and encouragement to me.

Acknowledgements

I am grateful to Gratien (husband), Dr Theresita (daughter), Franciscan Friar and Priest, Dr Prins Casinader (brother), Therese (mother-in-law) and Late Dr Lionel Joseph (father-in-law) for the support and encouragement they have given to me.

My profound gratitude to Professor Peter Hoskin, Professor of clinical oncology, Mount Vernon Cancer Centre, Northwood and Christie Hospital, Manchester for writing the foreword for my book.

I am also grateful to the specialist palliative care team, psychology team and Information & Technology team (in particular Mr Alex Copeland) of Lister Hospital, Stevenage for their support to me.

About the Book

Moved by a patient's severe cancer pain, I changed my career from cardiology into this field. This book is a product of my years of experience and knowledge in complex cancer pain management. It aims to enable the clinician with excellence and empathy in caring for these patients. The pathophysiology of pain is matched with pharmacology. Integrating pain management with oncology can improve quality and quantity of patients' lives. The book also explains the phenomenon of *opioid induced hyper-algesia*. In essence, this book endeavours to provide the clinician with a holistic understanding and management of *the pain of cancer*.

The Author

Foreword

Despite substantial advances in the treatment of cancer in the last decade sadly many patients suffer pain both due to progressive cancer and the complications of treatment. This may present in specialist oncology units, general hospital settings and in the community and thus knowledge of the complex phenomenon of 'cancer pain' is essential for all professions caring for patients with cancer. This practical guide to the management of cancer pain is a valuable resource addressing this need and is written for all those managing patients with cancer.

It includes important background information on the pathophysiology and psychology of cancer pain which is essential to understanding the unique characteristics of pain in this setting and its impact on the patient and their family. This is complemented by chapters on the pharmacology of complex pain management, modern analgesic use and the role of non- pharmacological treatments. The clinical scenarios towards the end of this chapter bring the theory into real life with examples of complex pain in patients with cancer and its effective management. Many patients receiving end of life care will also have significant pain problems and the final chapter addressing cancer pain in the dying patient offers valuable insights into effective pain management in this setting.

Written by a practising specialist in palliative care faced daily with such patients, both in the general hospital and specialist cancer centre setting, the opportunity to share in the author's experience and compassion for those patients in her care gives this book added value.

'The Pain of Cancer' should be an essential read for all doctors and nurses in frontline medicine who will day to day be faced with patients having complex pain problems related to cancer. Armed with the concepts and theory of pain management, embellished by real life practical examples contained within this book they will have increased confidence to provide effective pain management. Most importantly patients facing the despair of pain associated with cancer will have access to effective pain control.

Peter Hoskin
Northwood and Manchester
July 2022

Contents

Chapter 1 – Introduction 11

Chapter 2 – Understanding Cancer Pain 18

Chapter 3 – Typical Cancer Pain Syndromes 25

Chapter 4 – Patho-Physiology of Complex Cancer Pain 31

Chapter 5 – Pharmacology of Complex Cancer Pain Management 46

Chapter 6 – Psychology of Cancer Pain 76

Chapter 7 – Non-Pharmacological Approach to Cancer Pain Management 81

Chapter 8 – Managing Cancer Pain In the Dying Patient 86

References 91

Chapter 1
INTRODUCTION

Pain is an unpleasant sensory physical and emotional experience caused by actual or potential tissue damage or described in terms of such damage (Ref. 1). It is therefore a *whole person* experience. Pain was traditionally considered as a protective symptom warning the individual of a danger and potentially enabling escape from it or necessitating rest and healing (Ref. 4). However, in cancer, the pain often signifies a negative and hopeless meaning to the individual without enabling escape.

Cancer pain is complex in nature. In many instances it has a predominant neuropathic pain component caused by tumour infiltration. The tumour initially compresses and eventually infiltrates the adjacent neural sheath (Ref. 5). Tumour induced nerve injury as with other causes, sets in motion a cascade of abnormal and heightened electrical activity in the nervous system which travels right up to the somatic sensory cerebral cortex (Ref. 3).

The patient with cancer pain tends to undergo a lonely experience despite having family and friends. The need for different modalities of treatment such as surgery, chemotherapy, radiotherapy or immunotherapy and their adverse effects despite best efforts by the treating team, can create a sense of apprehension. This can be compounded by the fear of possible future tumour recurrence. Therefore, the patient can experience an exhausting, physical and emotional cancer journey which can compound the overall pain perception (Ref. 31). The clinician's empathy can provide comfort.

Pain perception and emotional state are crucially inter- linked in the overall pain experience. Existing anxiety or a depressive personality can impact on the patient's coping mechanisms. *Flash-back memories* of severe cancer pain in family or friends in the past, or its negative public perception, can contribute to the patient's own pain experience.

The site of cancer pain can also influence the pain experience. Rectal cancer infiltrating the pre-sacral nerve plexus can lead to severe pain that can be embarrassing and result in social isolation. The unremitting nocturnal neuropathic pain of pancreatic cancer infiltrating the coeliac nerve plexus can result in insomnia, consequent day time drowsiness and impact on the patient's coping strategies. It is often known that the patient suffers total distress, referred to as *total pain*.

Pain perception is multi-dimensional but ultimately influenced by the 'top-down' influence from the brain. Pain has sensory, emotive and cognitive components. The higher the intellect, greater is the *suffering* due to the cognitive, evaluative component which tends to analyse the pain (Ref. 3).

The Limbic system which is the core of the brain plays a crucial role in the affective, emotional pain experience. The *Amygdala* which is a part of this system is known to be associated with *anticipatory pain* linking past experience and memories with the present (Ref. 3).

In complex cancer pain there are often intermittent episodes of severe, *'crisis'* pain which can be emotionally very distressing and can potentially trigger self-harm. Their transient nature can lead to suspicion and disbelief by professionals. This can result in distrust, compounding the lonely and fearful experience of the patient. It is of vital importance that a trusting, compassionate professional-patient partnership is established from the start of the pain management process.

A confusing phenomenon yet not widely recognised is *'opioid induced hyper-algesia'* which results from rapid opioid dose escalation performed with the aim of controlling severe pain. This paradoxical phenomenon of worsening pain with increasing opioid doses is known to be caused by central hyper-excitation process which is linked to Glutamate action on NMDA (N-Methyl-D-Aspartate) receptors. Vigilance and timely recognition are crucial for prevention of this inadvertently caused vicious therapeutic situation (Ref. 10, 11, 12).

The challenge of controlling complex cancer pain is also due to the inevitable requirement for using carefully selected poly- pharmacological agents. This aims to provide *analgesic synergy* optimising analgesia while minimising medication induced toxicity since smaller drug doses are utilised.

Drug induced adverse effects, notably anti-muscarinic effects of Tricyclic anti-depressant drugs used in cancer pain management, can compound the adverse effects of opioids especially constipation and dry mouth. The recently highlighted adverse effect, namely QT-c prolongation (corrected QT interval on electrocardiogram) requires vigilance as it can lead to life threatening cardiac arrhythmias and even sudden, unexpected death (Ref. 17).

Effective and safe analgesic management enables timely and efficient oncological management. It will be evident that the cancer patient's quality and quantity of life can be concurrently improved (Ref. 2, 31). A multidisciplinary team approach to cancer pain management is very beneficial both to the patient and to the professionals.

The pain of cancer requires excellence in clinical management and empathy in care of the patient.

References:

1. International association for the study of pain-IASP
2. Saarto T. Palliative care and oncology: the case for early integration. *Eur J Palliative Care*. 2014; 21: 109
3. Melzack R, Wall P D. The challenge of pain 2008. Penguin Books Limited
4. Lynch M E, Craig K D, Peng P W H. Clinical pain management: a practical guide: 2011 Blackwell Publishing Limited
5. Hoskin and Makin. Oncology for Palliative Medicine: 1998 Oxford medical publications
10. Mercadante S, Arcuri E. Hyperalgesia and opioid switching. *Am J Hospice Palliative Care* 2005. 22: 291-4

11. Angst M S, Clark J D. Opioid induced hyperalgesia: a qualitative systematic review. Anaesthesiology 2006. 104: 570-87

12. Fallon M. Opioid induced hyperalgesia: fact or fiction? : *Palliative Medicine* 2008. 22: 5-6

17. Wilcock A, Howard P, Charlesworth S. *Palliative care formulary* 7. Pharmaceutical Press, 2020

31. Greer S, Joseph M. Palliative Care: A Holistic Discipline. *Integrative cancer therapies* 2015; 1-5

Chapter 2

UNDERSTANDING CANCER PAIN

The clinician is called upon to exercise clinical vigilance, understand the characteristics and expectancy for pain flare following oncological therapies such as radiotherapy and immunotherapy. In addition, the emotional distress associated with cancer pain and the effects on family and friends requires utmost empathy from the clinician.

Clinical vigilance

Recurrent pain in the tonsillar region with radiation to the ear without evidence of localised infection requires careful examination and timely specialist referral, as it can signify a tumour in the head and neck region (Ref. 5, 6, 7).

Un-resolving ipsilateral shoulder pain, particularly with radiation down the inner arm, can be due to an apical lung cancer (often known as 'Pancoast tumour') infiltrating the lower cord of the brachial plexus (Ref. 5, 6, 7).

Unremitting lumbar backache worse during lying down at night requiring the patient to sit up, lean forward in bed and use rocking movements to find relief is quite ominous as it can signify pain arising from a retro-peritoneal organ, such as the pancreas, or from retro-peritoneal para-aortic lymphadenopathy (Ref. 5, 6, 7).

Pain in the rectum resulting in a constant sensation to pass a stool or requiring frequent change of sitting position in order to ease the pain is suspicious of a rectal tumour infiltrating the meso-rectal nerve plexus (Ref. 5, 6, 7).

In a patient with cancer, sudden severe pain in the spine with exacerbation by any form of straining should alert the clinician to the possibility of spinal metastases. There may be radicular pain in the form of 'girdle pain' along the rib cage from thoracic spinal metastases. Similarly, sciatic pain can originate from lumbar or sacral spinal metastases (Ref. 30).

Spinal pain getting worse can imply thecal impingement by tumour preceding spinal cord compression. Worsening weight bearing pain in the hip can signify an impending fracture of the neck of femur from a large lytic metastasis. These clinical suspicions can enable timely management (Ref. 30).

Clinical characteristics

Complex cancer pain often has a neuropathic causation (ref: 4). Nerve fibre infiltration pain may not be directly evident on clinical grounds but analysis of the imaging helps to identify it. The patient often describes three different components of pain. A constant pain likened to an ache with a *vice like* quality, severe, intermittent *'crisis'* pain episodes described in terms of stabbing, electric current or burning and *nocturnal pain* disturbing the patient's sleep (Ref. 19, 20). These descriptions are important to ascertain carefully as they have treatment implications. With appropriate analgesics, the constant pain often reduces in its intensity, while the frequency and not the intensity of the *'crisis'* pain episodes that diminishes. Finally the nocturnal pain becomes less prominent. Synergistic pharmacological management can reduce the three pain components, as explained in chapter 5.

Pain flare following radiotherapy

Radiotherapy often causes initial inflammation and oedema for a few days. This process can result in a flare up of the tumour pain. The patient needs to be reassured that this is temporary and eventual pain relief is often obtained after a few weeks.

Following spinal radiotherapy, steroids are often continued for a week before dose reduction, in order to reduce this initial inflammation and to thereby protect the underlying spinal cord.

Equally, additional analgesics would be required during this initial post -radiotherapy period.

Pain flare following immunotherapy

Immunotherapy acts by increasing inflammation of the tumour in its attempt to control it. Hence it is understandable that following immunotherapy the patient may experience worsening of pain at least for a few weeks. The clinician needs to increase the analgesia temporarily and reassure the patient.

Empathy

While understanding the clinical aspects of cancer pain, the clinician needs to show utmost empathy to the patient. The fear of the unknown factors such as eventual benefit from oncological therapies, and adverse effects of treatment can make the overall pain experience worse. The requirement for opioid analgesics with their side effects and the stigma still attached to them with regard to addiction can leave the patient feeling helpless in the cancer journey (Ref. 31).

Key chapter summary points

- Pain characteristics of different cancer sites should alert clinical suspicion
- Complex cancer pain has a neuropathic component, often with three different descriptions

- Vigilance is required for the initial pain flare following radiotherapy or immunotherapy
- Successful cancer pain management requires clinical excellence and empathy

References:

4. Lynch M E, Craig K D, Peng P W H. Clinical pain management: a practical guide: 2011 Blackwell *Publishing* Limited
5. Hoskin and Makin. Oncology for Palliative Medicine: 1998 Oxford medical publications
6. Souhami and Tobias. Cancer and its management: 1987 Blackwell Scientific Publications
7. Davis M, Walsh D. cancer pain syndromes. *Euro. J. Pall. Care. 2000; 7(6)*
19. Bennett M. Neuropathic pain. Oxford university press, 2006
20. Rayment *et al*. Neuropathic cancer pain: prevalence, severity, analgesia and impact from European palliative care research collaborative: *Palliative Medicine* 2013. 8: 27

30. Joseph M, Tayar R. Spinal cord compression requires early detection. *Eur J Palliative Care*. 2005; 12: 141-143.

31. Greer S, Joseph M. Palliative Care: A Holistic Discipline. *Integrative cancer therapies* 2015; 1-5.

Chapter 3

TYPICAL CANCER PAIN SYNDROMES

Cancer can result in a dreaded painful experience. The word cancer can lead to an expectation that pain would always feature in the trajectory of the illness which may not necessarily be the case. However, the clinician needs to be aware that there are certain cancers that would predictably lead to significant pain in the patient's cancer journey. We will explore these cancer pain syndromes (Ref. 5, 6, 7).

Head & Neck Tumours

Tumours of the head and neck can infiltrate the cranial nerves and result in neuropathic pain. Typical examples are pain felt over the face or the external ear (pinna) from an oral or pharyngeal cancer. The description of the pain alerts the clinician that it is predominantly neuropathic in nature. The patient may describe an intense painful sensation likened to 'face on fire'. A severe, persistent, unexplained earache may be an initial manifestation of an oral-pharyngeal cancer. Other examples are cancer of the tonsil, tongue, maxillary antrum, and laryngeal cancer among others.

Clinical recognition of this pain is crucial not only to implement a timely diagnostic path-way but also appropriate analgesic action plan.

Apical Lung cancer

Tumours arising from the apex of the lung are often known as 'Pancoast tumours' and they can infiltrate the brachial plexus and the first two ribs. Pain can be felt in the shoulder region or down the arm and forearm into the little finger. A typical dermatomal distribution of the pain becomes evident such as C5 or C8, T1. Weakness of the small muscles of the hand may be present.

These features require early detection and appropriate analgesic and therapeutic interventions.

Malignant Mesothelioma

Malignant Mesothelioma plaques can infiltrate the intercostal neuro-vascular bundle resulting in severe neuropathic pain in the chest wall which can be mistaken for acute cardiac pain. In addition, the close proximity of the tumour to the intercostal vascular bundle can result in erosion through the thin- walled intercostal vein predisposing to a bleed and rapid clinical deterioration. Pain escalation in malignant mesothelioma should alert the clinician to the potential for a rapid decline into the terminal stage. This complication is important with respect to preparation of the patient, family and staff members. Also importantly, following the patient's death, it is a legal requirement to inform the coroner for compensation purposes owing to Asbestos exposure.

Cancer of pancreas

Cancer of the pancreas can infiltrate the coeliac nerve plexus. Being a retro-peritoneal organ, the patient experiences characteristic pain felt in the upper lumbar or the epigastric region, worse at night while lying down which can result in insomnia. The pain prompts the patient to sit up, rock forwards and backwards in order to obtain some relief. This is known as 'Fowler's position'. The pain gradually becomes worse with time and is predominantly 'neuropathic' in nature. In addition, to the constant ache the patient often experiences intermittent, excruciating *'crisis'* pain episodes and nocturnal pain that can result in day-time exhaustion.

Timely detection is required for appropriate oncological and analgesic management.

Cancer of rectum

Rectal tumour can infiltrate the pre-sacral nerve plexus. This can result in severe neuropathic pain in the rectum, often described as an unpleasant feeling of 'needles' in this area or a constant sensation to defecate. This pain is known as *tenesmus* and the entire sensation can be embarrassing to the patient. There can be silent *suffering* as the patient can struggle to explain the pain to family or friends. It can result in social isolation, loneliness and despondency.

This pain requires a sensitive and empathetic approach to management.

Spinal metastases

Spinal metastases from any cancer can impinge on the exiting nerve roots. This can result in excruciating 'radicular pain'. Impingement of the thecal sac can lead to severe pain made worse by cough, sneeze or any attempted straining or movement of the spine. These features can pre-empt spinal cord compression or *cauda-equina* compression depending on the involved spinal level. Thoracic radicular pain is felt in a girdle distribution along the rib-cage while sciatic pain can result from lumbar or sacral spinal metastases. Recognition of the pain leads to appropriate analgesic management and timely referral to oncology or surgery for possible spinal cord compromise.

Key chapter summary points

- Cancer pain syndromes can be detected by their clinical characteristics
- These painful syndromes are predominantly neuropathic in nature

- Potential spinal cord compromise can be suspected from the pain description
- Recognition can lead to timely oncological and analgesic management

References

5. Hoskin and Makin. Oncology For Palliative Medicine: 1998 Oxford medical publications.
6. Souhami and Tobias. Cancer and its management: 1987 Blackwell Scientific Publications.
7. Davis M, Walsh D. cancer pain syndromes. *Euro. J. Pall. Care*.2000; 7(6).

Chapter 4

PATHO-PHYSIOLOGY OF COMPLEX CANCER PAIN

Pain is an unpleasant symptom with both physical and emotional distress, caused by actual or potential tissue damage (Ref. 1). The sensation of pain often originats as a protective reflex response to injury. However, in the clinical context of cancer, the pain becomes progressive and loses its protective meaning. On the contrary, it becomes mal-adaptive, instilling fear and harm with negative, adverse prognostic implications, adding to the overall distress experienced by the patient.

The pain of *cancer* is often complex and as such in about 50%, has a predominant neuropathic pain component (Ref. 4, 8, 19, 20). The transient, elusive yet severe, *'crisis'* pain episodes can lead to a sense of disbelief by the health- care professional, while additionally instilling a feeling of despondency in the patient. Furthermore, there is often a sub-optimal analgesic response to opioid therapy, making the situation worse (Ref. 16). The patient can suffer total distress also referred to as *total pain* and may become socially isolated. The situation can leave the caring professional feeling frustrated and helpless.

Patho-physiology of pain is very similar to that of seizures (Ref. 3, 18). There exists a complex, multi- mechanistic process in the final pan perception (Ref. 3). Understanding this process will enable the rationale for a carefully selected and appropriately introduced poly-pharmacological therapeutic management similar to the treatment of complex seizures (Ref. 15, 17, 18).

Peripheral neural mechanisms

Pain sensing neural structures are known as 'nociceptors'. They are present both in the periphery as well as in the visceral regions of the body. These are activated by tissue injury and sensed by several ion channels including acid sensing ion channels (ASICs), voltage- gated sodium channels, voltage- gated calcium channels and potassium channels, ATP- related purinergic receptors and a new group of receptors known as transient receptor potential (TRP) family (Ref. 4). TRP plays a crucial role in visceral injury including that arising from cancer.

From the nociceptors, primary afferent neurones originate, consisting of A-Delta and C-fibres. The former are thinly myelinated and conduct pain impulses faster than the latter which are un- myelinated. It is traditionally known that A-Delta nerve fibres transmit the immediate, sharp pain while the C-fibres transmit more diffuse pain (Ref. 3, 4).

In addition, there are A-Beta nerve fibres which are thickly myelinated and rapidly transmit non- painful stimuli such as mechanical or thermal sensations (Ref. 3, 4).

These nerve fibres have their cell bodies in the dorsal nerve root ganglion. The emerging nerve fibres from this ganglion, synapse with second order neurones in the dorsal horn of the spinal cord in the region known as 'substantia gelatinosa' (Ref. 3, 4, 8). Out of nearly ten parallel nerve fibres in the dorsal spinal horn, known as layers or laminae, 1,2 and 5 are involved in pain transmission. Layer 2 has inter-neurones which act locally and do not transmit pain impulses to the brain. About 10% of lamina 5 neurones project pain impulses to the brain via the anterior and lateral spino-thalamic tracts (Ref. 3, 4).

A-Beta nerve fibres synapse in laminae 3, 4 and transmit non-painful stimuli (Ref. 3, 4).

In 1965, Melzack and Wall proposed the *gate-control theory* (Ref. 3). They suggested the existence of a putative gate in the substantia gelatinosa of the spinal dorsal horn which can block in-coming pain impulses from the A-Delta and C-fibres by the fast conducting A-Beta fibres. This may explain the reason why rubbing a painful area can bring comfort and the analgesic mechanism of acupuncture and trans-cutaneous electrical nerve stimulation (TENS).

Central neural mechanisms

Ascending pain facilitating neural path-ways

The second order neurones arising from the dorsal spinal horn, travel centrally in the anterior and lateral spino-thalamic nerve tracts, all the way up-to the thalamus. The third order neurones arising from the thalamus, project to the somatic sensory cerebral cortex in the parietal lobe of the brain which is associated with sensory discrimination of pain (Ref. 3, 4).

The main excitatory, neuro-transmitter in the spino-thalamic tracts is glutamate, released by intra- cellular calcium ion influx, and acts on N-Methyl-D-Aspartate (NMDA) receptors. Hence drugs that inhibit the calcium ion entry into the nerve cells such as gabapentin or pregabalin, have the potential to reduce neuropathic pain (Ref. 15, 17, 18, 19, 20). Similarly, NMDA antagonists, such as ketamine is sometimes used to relieve uncontrolled severe neuropathic pain in cancer (Ref. 15, 17,18, 19, 20, 24).

Third order neurones from the thalamus also project to parts of the limbic system of the brain, namely, the insula and anterior cingulate cortex which are associated with the affective-motivational component of pain perception (Ref. 3).

Descending pain inhibitory neural path-ways

Some of the third -order neurones from the thalamus, project downwards to the rostral, ventro- medial medulla and are involved in descending pain modulation of spinal dorsal horn neurones (Ref. 3, 4). Similarly, neural path-ways descend from the cingulate gyrus through the mid-brain peri-aqueductal grey matter (known as the PAG), and pass through the nucleus raphae magnus of the medulla oblongata and decussate with the spinal dorsal horn neurones (Ref. 3, 4).

These neural path-ways depend on the mono-amine neuro-transmitters, primarily nor-epinephrine. Drugs that augment nor-epinephrine in the synaptic cleft such as the tri-cyclic anti-depressant drugs (for example, amitriptyline, nortriptyline) or serotonin and norepinephrine re-uptake inhibitors (for example, duloxetine) or pre-synaptic alpha-2 adrenoceptor antagonist (for example, mirtazapine) can therefore reduce pain by augmenting the descending pain inhibition which is now considered to be crucial in complex pain management (Ref. 3, 4).

Limbic- system influence on pain perception

The limbic system of the brain is known to influence pain, mood, appetite and sleep. Amygdala of the limbic- brain, is associated with the causation of *anticipatory pain* by connecting past experiences and memories with the present (Ref. 3). The hippocampus of the limbic-brain is known as the 'cognitive map' (Ref. 3). It can exert a positive influence on the *amygdala* by rationalising events. The cingulate cortex of the limbic-brain from where descending pain inhibitory path-ways can also commence, can be influenced positively by distraction and psychological therapies such as cognitive behavioural therapy (CBT).

'Gate control theory'

When Ronald Melzack and Patrick Wall proposed the *gate control theory* in 1965 (Ref. 3), they implied that this putative gate in the spinal dorsal horn can be closed by rapid incoming non-noxious stimuli such as mechanical, thermal and vibration, thereby reduce pain.

'Neuro-matrix theory'

With expanding knowledge in the 21st century, it became clear that the brain had the ultimate, overall control in the final pain perception. It explained the 'neuro-matrix theory' where an individual's past experiences, memories, beliefs, coping strategies and personal meaning of pain can collectively contribute to the eventual pain experience (Ref. 3).

Hence, the *neuro-matrix* theory expounds rather than replace the *gate control theory*.

Bio-chemical and cellular mechanisms involved in pain

In the conduction of nociceptive or painful signals, ion channels and neuro-transmitters are involved. The initial signalling is via the sensory neurone specific sodium channels which are followed by the voltage-gated calcium ion channels (Ref. 4). Activation of these channels leads to the release of excitatory neuro-transmitters, mainly glutamate which acts on NMDA receptors. Peptidergic neurones release excitatory neuro-transmitters, namely substance-P which acts on neurokinin 1 receptors and calcitonin gene related peptide (CGRP). Inhibition of these chemicals can form the basis of future analgesic adjuvants in complex pain management.

Peripheral sensitisation process

Pro-inflammatory mediators are released at the site of tissue injury. These among other are, namely, serotonin, glutamate, peptides such as substance-P, CGRP, bradykinin, lipids such as prostaglandins, cytokines such as interleukins as well as neuro-trophins. They lead to peripheral inflammation via a cascading process involving 2nd messengers and perpetuate the peripheral sensitisation process which reduces the threshold for activation of pain impulses (Ref. 4).

Central sensitisation process

In persistent pain situations such as *cancer* and in chronic pain situations such as fibromyalgia, long- term 'plastic' changes occur in the spinal dorsal horn and the brain. There is heightened spontaneous electrical activity, reduced activation thresholds and expansion in the size of the receptive fields which are a fraction of dermatomes (Ref. 3).

The mechanisms underlying the above process are thought to be among others, namely, NMDA activation, loss of inhibitory pain control also known as *dis-inhibition*, interaction between microglia, astrocytes and the spinal dorsal horn neurones and the paradoxical process of descending pain facilitation (Ref. 4).

With repeated nerve injury and persistence of pain, NMDA receptors are activated by the powerful excitatory neuro-transmitter, glutamate which is also implicated in memory formation (Ref. 4). Hence it is important to control pain before memory aggravates the pain experience.

In addition, the pain inhibitory processes are reversed and a shift occurs to an 'excitatory mode' after persistent injury. Inhibitory neuro-transmitters such as gamma-amino-butyric-acid, known as GABA and Glycine now become excitatory instead of inhibitory due to changes in the internal environment of the nervous system (Ref. 4).

Further-more, microglia interact with the spinal dorsal horn neurones and release chemicals among others, namely, interleukins and brain- derived neuro-trophic factors which enhance the central sensitisation process and contribute to persistent pain (Ref. 4). Astrocytes are thought to be involved in the maintenance rather than the induction of persistent pain (Ref. 4).

In addition, the usual pain inhibition via the mid-brain peri-aqueductal grey, known as the PAG and the rostro-ventral medulla (RVM) now begin to facilitate pain. NMDA activation, BDNF and microglial contribution are now thought to be involved in this process of descending pain facilitation (Ref. 4).

It is perceivable that pain perpetuation once started, continues unabated, leading to the distress suffered by the patient even after the original injury has healed. This may explain the mechanism behind *phantom limb pain* that is known to occur after the amputation of a severely painful limb.

The crucial features of this sensitisation process are clinically manifested in the form of *allodynia* in particular *tactile allodynia*, where gentle stroking of the painful area of skin exacerbates the pain and *hyper-algesia*, which means heightened pain (Ref. 3, 4, 8, 20).

Dimensions of human pain perception

Unlike animals, humans have a cognitive, evaluative component to pain perception (Ref. 3). They tend to analyse pain and unduly worry about its implications such as the possibility of *cancer* progression. This evaluative, analytical component adds to the discriminative and emotive aspects of pain perception. It is known that the higher the intellect, the greater is the overall suffering and pain experience. Understandably, health-care professionals are known to experience more pain than their non-health care counter-parts.

Factors influencing ultimate pain perception

THE PAIN OF CANCER

The brain ultimately decides the final pain perception. This is influenced by past memories of pain in family and friends, coping strategies, beliefs, expectations, life goals and family concerns. No two patients with the same *cancer* are likely to experience similar pain perception (Ref. 3, 8, 20).

This should be borne in mind when healthcare professionals try to control pain and it demands utmost empathy in caring in addition to clinical excellence in complex pain management (Ref. 31).

Key chapter summary points
- Complex pain is caused by a multi-mechanistic patho-physiology similar to that of seizure
- Ascending pain-facilitating path-ways via the spinothalamic nerve tracts are served by the excitatory neuro-transmitter, glutamate, which is triggered by calcium ion influx into the cell
- Descending pain-inhibitory neural pathways passing through the brainstem

and synapsing in the dorsal spinal horn, mainly require Norepinephrine in the synaptic clefts

- The limbic system of the brain is associated with pain, mood, appetite and sleep
- There are sensory, emotive and cognitive aspects to human pain perception
- The brain exerts an overall influence on the individual's ultimate pain perception

References

1. International association for the study of pain-IASP
3. Melzack R, Wall, P D. The challenge of pain 2008. Penguin Books Limited
4. Lynch M E, Craig K D, Peng P W H. Clinical pain anagement: a practical guide: 2011 Blackwell Publishing Limited
8. Leon-Casasola O A D. cancer pain: 2006; *Saunders Elsevier (www. Elsevier.com)*
15. Bennett M. palliative medications: drugs for neuropathic pain. *Euro. J. Pall. Care* 2010;17(4)

16. Dickenson A. The science of opioids. The 10th Annual Royal Marsden pain and opioid conference 2017
17. Wilcock A, Howard P, Charlesworth S. *Palliative care formulary 7.* Pharmaceutical Press, 2020
18. Smith H. Drugs for pain 2002: ISBN 1-56053-511-3
19. Bennett M. Neuropathic pain. Oxford university press, 2006
20. Rayment *et al.* Neuropathic cancer pain: prevalence, severity, analgesia and impact from European palliative care research collaborative: *Palliative Medicine* 2013. 8: 27
24. Prommer E. Ketamine for pain: an update for uses in palliative care. *J. palliative med.* 2012
31. Greer S, Joseph M. Palliative Care: A Holistic Discipline. *Integrative cancer therapies* 2015; 1-5

Chapter 5

PHARMACOLOGY OF COMPLEX CANCER PAIN MANAGEMENT

The pain of cancer is often complex and has a predominant neuropathic component (Ref. 4, 20). It is similar to seizure in its pathophysiology (ref. 3, 4, 8). Therefore, a multi-modal pharmacological management becomes necessary in most situations of complex cancer pain. This approach requires a careful therapeutic decision making process in order to achieve efficacy and safety of analgesic management. Hence, analgesic success relies on efficacy and safety.

Multi-modal pharmacological management

The therapeutic principle of *analgesic synergy* is the basis of multi-modal pharmacological management of complex *cancer* pain which as we know has a multi-mechanistic pathophysiology in its causation (Ref. 18, 19, 20). A step-wise introduction of an opioid, followed by a voltage-gated calcium-ion channel blocker and further followed if required, by the addition of a synaptic Norepinephrine enhancer often provides a useful, triangular analgesic synergy. This pharmacological method reduces the potential for inadvertent dose escalation of each analgesic. Synergy differs from combination effect since the overall benefit is not due to summation but rather an augmentation utilising different pharmacological mechanisms of action resulting in overall heightened analgesia. Smaller analgesic doses are enabled by the process of synergy which maximises efficacy and minimises medication toxicity.

Opioid:

Role

Opioids are effective analgesics for *cancer* pain relief (Ref. 16, 17, 18). They are known to act at spinal and supra-spinal levels. The analgesic ladder introduced by the world health ˙isation in the 1980s has three steps. in steps 2 and 3. Over-reliance on step 2 analgesics such as codeine used for mild to moderate pain can lead to delay and sub-optimal analgesia in *cancer* pain management. Furthermore, codeine is very constipating. An opioid from step 3 used for moderate to severe pain such as morphine is often required for timely and optimal analgesia in cancer.

Choice and safety

The choice of opioid used, depends primarily on the patient's renal function.

Morphine is the initial opioid of choice if the e-GFR (estimated glomerular filtration rate, which is an estimate of renal function) is greater than 30 millilitres (ml) per minute. If the e-GFR is less than 30ml per minute, oxycodone is likely to be safer. It is twice as potent as morphine as an analgesic but is more constipating. Appropriate analgesic and laxative dosage adjustments will be needed. Oxycodone should be avoided in significant liver impairment as it is primarily metabolised by the liver, unless the patient is in the dying stage and is comfortable on it. In significant renal impairment metabolites of morphine, mainly M3G (morphine 3 glucuronide' accumulate in the blood and can result in central nervous system toxicity.

If the e-GFR is less than 15ml per minute, alfentanil via a sub-cutaneous infusion may be safer. However, in this situation, small doses of oxycodone may be acceptable according to medication availability and clinician's experience.

In the presence of significant hepatic and renal impairment, the safest opioid analgesic would be alfentanil, since metabolites of morphine are excreted through the kidneys and oxycodone is metabolised by the liver. However, practicality, medication availability and clinician experience should be taken into account in deciding the safe and optimal choice of opioid.

Trans-dermal fentanyl opioid patch applied every 72 hours is useful when stable analgesia is achieved and in patients with head and neck cancers who have impaired swallowing.

Opioid toxicity

Opioid toxicity often manifests in the form of drowsiness, impaired cognition, myoclonic jerks which manifest as irregular jerks of the limbs, visual hallucinations which are often described as seeing *crawling insects* and very small pupils, provided a concurrent anti-muscarinic drug which dilates the pupils is not in use. The features of opioid toxicity can be subtle in early stages and may only manifest during periods of falling asleep or waking, known as the *hypnogogic state*. Respiratory depression occurs in the late stages of opioid toxicity.

Prior to any opioid dose increase in order to improve analgesia, opioid toxicity should be ruled out. Once it is safe to do so, the opioid dose is increased by 30% or 50%. If there is inadequate analgesia in the presence of opioid toxicity, a switch to an alternate opioid should be preferably undertaken with a dose reduction.

Unexplained opioid toxicity should prompt vigilance for the detection of impaired renal function. This can be due to the *cancer* or nephrotoxicity from concurrent use of adjuvant analgesic medications such as non-steroidal anti-inflammatory drugs.

Essential laxative use with opioid

A stool softener and a stimulant laxative should be co-prescribed with any opioid as constipation occurs universally with all opioids, with some more than with others. This need is because opioids result in hardening of intestinal luminal contents and reversal of peristalsis (*retro-peristalsis).*

Codeine and oxycodone are the most constipating opioids and fentanyl is least constipating.

Dosage guidance

Immediate release oral *morphine* solution (known as oramorph) at a dose of 5mg every 4 hours is a safe starting dose. In an out-patient setting, prescribing modified release *morphine* 15mg 12 hourly can be more pragmatic for use at home.

The equivalent dose of immediate release oxycodone oral solution would be 2.5mg every 4 hours.

The equivalent dose of fentanyl trans-dermal patch would be 12 micrograms per hour, applied every 72 hours.

The above dosages would be the starting doses of opioids for analgesia. Dose increase can be undertaken if required for improved analgesia, by 30%-50% provided there is no evidence of opioid toxicity. In frail, elderly patients, dosages should preferably be kept as low as possible.

It is safer not to exceed MORPHINE modified release dose of 60mg 12 hourly or its equivalent OXYCODONE modified release dose of 30mg 12 hourly or FENTANYL trans-dermal patch dose of 50microgram per hour applied every 72 hours. These modest opioid doses will be enabled by the careful use of analgesic synergy as explained later. It is worthy of note that higher opioid doses have the potential to result in *opioid induced hyperalgesia* as explained later in this chapter.

Exceptionally higher opioid doses may be required particularly for severe uncontrolled pain in the terminal, dying stage of cancer.

Voltage- gated calcium ion channel blocker:

Role

Both gabapentin and pregabalin act on the alpha- 2 delta sub-unit of the voltage-gated calcium- ion channels and reduce the calcium -ion influx into the neuronal cell (Ref. 15, 17, 18, 19). This reduction of intra-cellular calcium ions results in reduced glutamate release. Glutamate is a powerful, excitatory neuro-transmitter which acts on NMDA (N-Methyl D- Aspartate) receptors and responsible for the central sensitisation process which is the primary cause of complex pain in cancer. Hence these drugs will reduce this process and thereby reduce pain. Gabapentin or pregabalin will provide analgesic synergy with opioid enabling low doses of these analgesic drugs.

Choice and safety

Pregabalin attaches more avidly to the receptors on the calcium- ion channels than gabapentin and it also has a linear pharmaco-kinetic profile. Hence dose increase improves analgesic efficacy unlike with gabapentin whose analgesic action tends to reach a plateau phase after some weeks of use.

Both gabapentin and pregabalin require adequate renal function for their safe use. In significant renal impairment, smaller drug doses should be used and dose titration performed slowly.

Neurotoxicity from these drugs can manifest in the form of giddiness, drowsiness and ataxia (unsteady gait). Nystagmus detected on lateral conjugate gaze can be used as an indirect proxy sign which can pre-empt the development of neurotoxicity from gabapentin or pregabalin. They can also cause fluid retention resulting in ankle oedema and potentially worsen congestive cardiac failure.

Dosage guidance

Gabapentin is started at a dose of 300mg at night and gradually up-titrated after 3 days to 300mg morning and evening and further increased after 3 days if required and tolerated to 300mg three times daily, provided renal function is satisfactory.

In significant renal impairment, or in frailty, it is safer to commence 100mg at night and gradually up- titrate after 3 days to 100mg morning and evening with further gradual increase as required, maintaining overall smaller doses.

Pregabalin is preferably commenced at a dose of 25mg morning and evening, unlike the previous higher starting dose regime, in order to reduce the risk of neurotoxicity and thus preserve medication compliance. It is up-titrated, preferably in a step-wise manner after 2 days to 25 mg morning and 50mg in the evening. After a further 2 days, if the patient is tolerating it but requires further analgesia, the dose can be increased to 50mg morning and evening. Further gradual increases can be undertaken according to analgesic need and tolerability.

In significant renal impairment, the safer starting dose would be 25mg in the evening with even more gradual dose titration maintaining smaller overall dose.

In general, it is safer not to exceed PREGABALIN 150mg BD dose or its equivalent

GABAPENTIN 600mg TDS since higher doses are unlikely to provide additional analgesic benefit but are likely to result in neuro-toxicity.

Synaptic norepinephrine enhancer:

Role

Analgesics in the class of tricyclic anti-depressant drugs, serotonin and norepinephrine re-uptake inhibitors, pre-synaptic alpha- 2 adrenoceptor antagonists, increase the norepinephrine in the synaptic clefts (Ref. 17, 18, 19). The brain-stem pain-inhibitory neural pathways require norepinephrine as the primary neurochemical for their action. Therefore, any drug that enhances norepinephrine in the synaptic cleft has the potential to provide analgesia by augmenting pain inhibition which is now considered to be the most important mechanism in pain management (Ref. 3). They provide useful analgesic synergy with opioid and voltage- gated calcium-ion channel blocker enabling the use of smaller doses.

Choice and safety
Tricyclic anti-depressant drugs (TCAs)

TCAs, namely amitriptyline or nortriptyline are very effective in providing analgesic synergy with opioid and voltage-gated calcium-ion channel blocker in complex *cancer* pain management.

However, they result in significant anti-muscarinic adverse effects, notably constipation which adds to that caused by opioid. They can also cause dry mouth, urinary hesitancy or retention and blurred vision from pupillary dilatation which can exacerbate close-angle glaucoma. Nortriptyline, being a secondary amine TCA, unlike amitriptyline which is a tertiary amine TCA, is considered to possess a less severe anti-muscarinic burden.

TCAs are known to exacerbate cardiac conduction abnormalities and postural hypotension. They can prolong the QTc (corrected QT) interval, predisposing to ventricular arrhythmias and even a sudden death.

Another rare yet serious adverse effect is serotonin syndrome, particularly when used with opioids in high doses. This manifests as neuro-muscular irritability such as muscle twitching, autonomic dysfunction such as altered blood pressure, pyrexia, sweating and mental abnormalities such as agitation. Vigilance and recognition of this life threatening *albeit* rare adverse effect, discontinuation of offending drug/s, fluid resuscitation and cooling measures are crucial to save life.

Serotonin and norepinephrine re-uptake inhibitor (SNRI):

Duloxetine and Venlafaxine belong to this group.

Venlafaxine is used in severe depression under psychiatric-specialist supervision and hence understandably not used in complex *cancer* pain management.

Duloxetine is used in diabetic peripheral neuropathy, but it can be used to control complex cancer pain, enabling analgesic synergy with opioid and voltage-gated calcium-ion channel blocker.

However, SNRIs do have the potential to result in hypertension, and serotonin syndrome.

Hence careful clinical supervision and vigilance are required.

Pre-synaptic alpha-2 adrenoceptor antagonist:

Mirtazapine which belongs to this group has the potential to improve pain, mood, appetite and sleep (Ref. 21, 22, 23). It can be useful in providing analgesic synergy with opioid and voltage-gated calcium-ion channel blocker in complex cancer pain management. Initial drowsiness tends to improve with up-ward dose-titration as anti-histaminergic effect gives way to dopaminergic effect. Improved appetite can be useful in cancer induced anorexia but weight gain can worsen diabetic control.

Dosage guidance

Amitriptyline or Nortriptyline is commenced at a dose of 10mg at night and can be increased if needed and tolerated, after 48 hours, to 20mg at night.

Duloxetine is started at a dose of 30mg at night, provided renal function is satisfactory. If necessary, for further analgesia, after 3 nights, the dose can be increased to 60mg at night.

Mirtazapine is started at a dose of 15mg at night and increased after 3 nights to 30mg at night, provided renal function is satisfactory. After 10 days, maximum dose of 45mg at night can be used if required and tolerated.

Triangular analgesic synergy

It will be evident that opioid, voltage-gated calcium-ion channel blocker and a synaptic norepinephrine enhancer introduced in a step-wise manner can together form useful, triangular analgesic synergy in complex *cancer* pain management. This synergy is aimed to improve analgesia and prevent rapid dose escalation of each analgesic, thus minimising adverse drug effects. Importantly, it can prevent the serious phenomenon of *opioid induced hyper-algesia,* described later.

They are introduced in a step-wise manner while attempting to maintain smaller doses of each drug. They have the potential to maximise analgesic efficacy and minimise medication induced toxicity.

THE PAIN OF CANCER

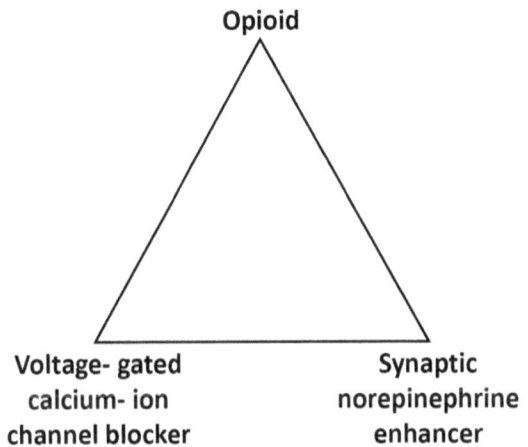

Dual analgesic synergy

Opioid and a voltage-gated calcium-ion channel blocker can form useful dual synergy in the initial stages of cancer pain management.

Tapentadol by possessing *mu* opioid agonistic effect and norepinephrine re-uptake inhibitor effect can provide dual analgesic synergy but is currently reserved for resistant chronic pain in the non- palliative care setting.

Opioid-induced hyper-algesia (OIH)

This is a serious phenomenon caused by rapid opioid dose escalation performed with the aim of controlling severe pain (Ref. 9, 10, 11, 12, 13, 14). The high opioid dose enhances the central sensitisation process, thereby exacerbating the pain. Recognition of OIH and opioid dose reduction are crucial in order to avert this vicious circle. OIH can be present with or without clinical features of opioid toxicity (Ref. 12).

The use of analgesic synergy which prevents rapid and inadvertent opioid dose escalation can reduce the potential for the development of OIH. If pregabalin or gabapentin is introduced in the presence of OIH, serious respiratory depression can occur (MHRA alert 2021).

The role of steroid

Dexamethasone is a powerful steroid which can reduce peri-tumour oedema, inflammation and oedema around nerve sheaths, thereby improve analgesia (Ref. 17).

Dosage guidance

Dexamethasone 8mg daily is useful as a starting dose with adequate gastro-duodenal protection with a proton pump inhibitor or Histamine-2 antagonist. The dose can be reduced after 5 days to the smallest effective dose. Precautions in order to protect steroid safety are required including prevention of proximal myopathy and vigilance for increased blood glucose and the development of oral candidiasis. A steroid card outlining the steroid plan should be provided to the patient in order to aid clinical care in other settings.

The role of non-steroidal anti-inflammatory drug

In cancer pain situations with a significant inflammatory component, Naproxen can be used (not with steroid) initially 250mg twice daily or 500mg once daily with gastric protection (Ref. 17, 18).

The role of benzodiazepines:

In complex pain situations, *dis-inhibition* which is a process that dampens the pain inhibitory path- ways exists (Ref. 3). Benzodiazepines and relaxation techniques can improve this process and result in better analgesia. In addition, they are agonists of gamma-amino-butyric-acid (GABA) which is a powerful inhibitory neurotransmitter which can reduce the excitatory component of pain facilitation.

Clonazepam

Clonazepam being a benzodiazepine can provide relaxation and GABA agonistic effect which can provide further analgesic synergy in uncontrolled complex cancer pain (Ref. 17, 18). It can also improve sleep. Since sedation can limit its use, smaller increments are required.

Dosage guidance

Clonazepam is commenced at a dose of 250 microgram at night and up-titrated after 2 nights to 500 microgram at night if tolerated and provided there is no significant hepatic or renal impairment. Further gradual up-titration can be undertaken if required up to a maximum of 2mg daily.

The role of combined opioid therapy

In exceptional situations where pain control is proving difficult despite optimal opioid and co- analgesic synergistic adjuvant therapy as described above, a small dose of an additional opioid methadone can be carefully considered at a dose of 2.5mg at night (Ref. 17, 26) in a supervised setting.

In the dying patient with cancer, addition of another opioid via a continuous sub-cutaneous infusion also commonly referred to as a *syringe driver* together with an existing trans-dermal opioid is considered as acceptable therapeutic practice (Ref. chapter 8) in order to maximise comfort.

The role of NMDA antagonists:

NMDA (N-Methyl D-Aspartate) antagonists block the action of glutamate, the powerful excitatory neuro-transmitter implicated in central sensitisation process contributing to complex pain (refer to chapter 4).

In uncontrolled pain or in the situation of OIH, NMDA antagonist provides useful anti-hyper-algesic effect, reducing the central sensitisation process and thereby improving opioid analgesia. Hence, it is advisable to reduce the concurrent opioid dose when commencing an NMDA antagonist in order to avoid opioid toxicity (Ref. 19).

Ketamine

Ketamine is in this group (Ref. 19, 24). However, it can result in distressing, psycho-mimetic adverse effects, manifested as confusion, dissociation, and delirium. It can worsen seizures and psychiatric disorders. Being a positive chronotropic and inotropic drug, it can also result in hypertension. It can increase intra-cranial pressure. These cautions should be observed when considering the use of Ketamine. Clonazepam (a benzodiazepine) or haloperidol (an anti-psychotic drug) should be used with Ketamine in order to prevent psycho-mimetic adverse effects. For the above reasons, Ketamine is initiated in a supervised clinical setting in order to ensure patient safety.

Dosage guidance

Ketamine is preferably commenced via a single continuous sub-cutaneous infusion at a dose of 100 mg over 24 hours, diluted in normal saline. If tolerated and required for improved analgesia, the dose can be increased daily by 50mg or 100 mg up- to a maximum dose of 400 mg daily (Ref. 19).

When ketamine sub-cutaneous infusion is converted to oral preparation, the dose is halved after about two days, since oral hepatic by-pass process results in the conversion to nor-ketamine which is a more potent analgesic than the parent drug (Ref. 19).

Analgesic choice via gastrostomy tubes

Oral analgesic solutions which are safe to be administered via feeding tubes should be used.

With regard to a synaptic norepinephrine enhancer, a good choice in keeping with feeding tube safety and cost-efficacy would be amitriptyline oral solution (25mg in 5ml), starting with 10mg at night and up-titrating gradually after 48 hours to 20mg at night. In this regard, nortriptyline oral solution would be unnecessarily expensive. Equally, mirtazapine oro-dispersible preparation has the potential to occlude the feeding tube and the oral solution would be unnecessarily expensive.

With regard to a voltage-gated calcium-ion channel blocker, pregabalin oral solution can be safely administered via a feeding tube. Alternatively the contents of the pregabalin capsule can be dissolved in warm water and administered through a feeding tube and flushed well afterwards.

Clinical case scenarios exemplifying safe and effective analgesic synergy in action

Scenario 1

Severe pain due to peripheral sensory neuropathy preventing on-going use of chemotherapy;

Safe and effective analgesia obtained with the following triangular analgesic synergy, enabling continuation of chemotherapy:

- Oxycodone modified release 20mg 12 hourly

- Gabapentin 600mg TDS
- Mirtazapine 30mg nocte

Scenario 2

Tumour spread to the chest wall and existing fibromyalgia resulting in significant, predominant neuropathic pain;

Evidence of opioid induced hyper-algesia on large dose of Oxycodone modified release;

Borderline opioid toxicity, suspicious neuro-muscular irritability with duloxetine and ataxia with high dose pregabalin were clinically evident; clonazepam was already in place for associated anxiety;

Eventual safe and reasonably effective analgesia was achieved with the following quadruple analgesic synergy enabling a successful discharge home:

- Oxycodone modified release 30mg 12 hourly (gradual significant dose reduction to this dose)
- Pregabalin 150mg BD (dose reduction to this dose)

- Mirtazapine 45mg nocte (up-titrated to this dose & discontinued duloxetine)
- Clonazepam 1.5mg nocte (gentle increase to this dose)

Further examples of successful analgesic synergy

Brachial plexus infiltration pain:

Successful triangular analgesic synergy with immediate release morphine 5mg QDS, gabapentin 600mg TDS, mirtazapine 30mg at night;

Successful dual analgesic synergy with modified release morphine 15mg 12 hourly, mirtazapine 30mg at night and steroid dexamethasone 4mg morning;

Head and neck cancer pain:

Successful triangular analgesic synergy with transdermal fentanyl patch 25microgram per hour applied every 72 hours, pregabalin 50mg TDS, mirtazapine 30mg at night;

Pain from lumbar spinal degenerative disease in the context of cancer:

Successful triangular analgesic synergy with modified release oxycodone 30mg 12 hourly, gabapentin 300mg TDS and mirtazapine 30mg at night;

Successful triangular analgesic synergy with modified release oxycodone 30mg 12 hourly, pregabalin 150mg BD, mirtazapine 45mg at night.

Pain from perineal tissue injury following curative cancer therapy:

Successful dual analgesic synergy achieved with transdermal fentanyl patch 50microgram per hour applied every 72 hours, pregabalin 50mg morning, 50mg mid-day and 75mg at night.

Pain from meso-rectal tumour infiltration:

Successful triangular analgesic synergy achieved with modified release oxycodone 5mg 12 hourly, pregabalin 50mg TDS and mirtazapine 30mg at night.

Key chapter summary points
- Complex cancer pain requires careful, multi-modal pharmacological management in keeping with its complex patho-physiology
- Useful triangular analgesic synergy is produced by the step-wise introduction of an opioid, voltage-gated calcium-ion channel blocker and a synaptic norepinephrine enhancer
- Analgesic synergy can be improved further if required, with the benzodiazepine, clonazepam
- Opioid-induced hyper-algesia, requires vigilance and timely opioid dose reduction. Co- analgesic adjuvant use will help to prevent this serious condition
- Pharmacological ceiling doses for safety should always be borne in mind
- Analgesic synergy maximises efficacy and minimises medication induced toxicity
- Analgesic success relies on efficacy and medication safety

References

3. Melzack R, Wall P D. The challenge of pain 2008: Penguin Books Limited

4. Lynch M E, Craig K D, Peng P W H. Clinical pain management: a practical guide: 2011 Blackwell Publishing Limited

8. Leon-Casasola O A D. *cancer* pain: 2006; *Saunders Elsevier (www.elsevier.com)*

9. Mao J. Opioid induced abnormal pain sensitivity: Implications in clinical opioid therapy. Pain 2002. 100: 213-7

10. Mercadante S, Arcuri E. Hyperalgesia and opioid switching. *Am J Hospice Palliative Care* 2005. 22: 291-4

11. Angst M S, Clark J D. Opioid induced hyperalgesia: a qualitative systematic review. Anaesthesiology 2006. 104: 570-87

12. Fallon M. Opioid induced hyperalgesia: fact or fiction? : *Palliative Medicine* 2008. 22: 5-6

13. Bannister K. Opioid induced hyperalgesia-lost in translation? The 10th Annual Royal Marsden pain and opioid conference 2017

14. Virani F. Opioid induced hyperalgesia. *BMJ specialist palliative care* 2020
15. Bennett M. palliative medication: drugs for neuropathic pain. *Euro. J. Pall. Care* 2010; 17 (4)
16. Dickenson A. The science of opioids: The 10th Annual Royal Marsden pain and opioid conference 2017
17. Wilcock A, Howard P, Charlesworth S. *Palliative care formulary 7.* Pharmaceutical Press, 2020
18. Smith H. Drugs for pain 2002: ISBN 1-56053-511-3
19. Bennett M. Neuropathic pain: Oxford university press, 2006
20. Rayment *et al.* Neuropathic *cancer* pain: prevalence, severity, analgesia and impact from European palliative care research collaborative: *Palliative Medicine* 2013. 8: 27

21. Theobald D E, Kirsh K L, Holtsclan E *et al.* An open-label cross-over trial of mirtazapine (15mg & 30mg) in cancer patients with pain and other distressing symptoms. *J. Pain Symptom Management* 2002. 23: 442-447

22. Montgomery S A. Safety of mirtazapine: a review. *Int. clin. psych. pharm.* 1995. 10:4, 37-45

23. Boer T D. The pharmacologic profile of mirtazapine: *J. CLIN. Psychiatry 1996;* 57 (suppl. 4)

24. Prommer E. Ketamine for pain: an update for uses in palliative care. *J. palliative. Med.* 2021. 4: 474-83

26. Reddy A *et al.* Dual opioid therapy using methadone as a co-analgesic: *Expert Opin. Drug Saf.* 2015; 14 (1); 181-183

Glossary

MHRA: Medicines and Healthcare products Regulatory Agency

Chapter 6

PSYCHOLOGY OF CANCER PAIN

Cancer can cause one of the worst pain experiences in humans and understandably is dreaded. It can be as severe as post-traumatic pain. The uncertainty of outcome, and the fear of *cancer* progression, can contribute to the overall pain perception and resultant *suffering* (Ref. 31).

The influence of the Limbic system

AMYGDALA which is a part of the limbic system of the brain can provide 'affective bias' by connecting past painful memories with the present (Ref. 3). The patient may recall severe pain episodes which happened years previously in family or friends. The memory can return as 'flash- backs'. The patient may wrongly assume that the pain signifies cancer progression or even impending death.

Another part of the Limbic system, known as the *HIPPOCAMPUS*, provides a 'cognitive map' (Ref. 3). It evaluates the meaning of pain. The higher the intellect, the greater will be this evaluative component. Referred pain may be wrongly evaluated by the patient as due to cancer progression.

These processes can add to the overall pain experience.

Fear of dying

Patients mostly tend to fear the dying stage. They may have young family, with unfinished tasks and unattained goals in life. The severity of cancer pain may heighten this anxiety. Fear of dying in pain is a natural concern for every human. The patient might fear that the clinician may have exhausted all options for successful pain management.

Quality of life and analgesic adverse effects

Patients often prefer to be cognitively unaffected by pain management in order to undertake their daily tasks. Therefore, they may prefer to tolerate some degree of pain rather than increase the opioids. The clinician needs to respect this wish. Shared decision making with the patient is important with regard to every aspect of pain management.

Opioids inevitably result in constipation. This side effect ought to be guarded against by the judicious use of appropriate laxatives from the initiation of opioid therapy in *cancer* pain management.

Patients who are prone to migraine, vestibular disorders, or motion sickness are very likely to experience nausea and vomiting with the initiation of opioids. Therefore the clinician needs to be aware of the patient's history and commence appropriate anti-emetics from the initiation of opioid treatment in this group of patients. Failure to do so can lead to poor compliance with the opioid, resulting in uncontrolled pain.

Some patients fear that controlling *cancer* pain can mask its progression. This should be carefully explored with the patient and appropriate reassurance given.

Certain religious beliefs may result in the patient attributing the pain to atonement for sins. This concept should be sensitively explored and appropriate religious support should be sought.

The stigma attached to *MORPHINE*

Morphine is a very effective analgesic which has long been used successfully in cancer pain management. Unfortunately the word *morphine* is often associated with *cancer* by the public. The main issue here is not the *morphine* but the unfortunate assumption of *cancer progression*.

Morphine is safe when used carefully by clinicians. The diverted fear of *cancer* progression should be sensitively and empathetically explored by the clinician and appropriate reassurance given.

Empathy by the clinician

The clinician needs to practise sensitivity and empathy when caring for a patient with cancer. Understanding the patient's wishes and fears can lead to a good patient-clinician partnership. Unresolved psychological issues can add to the suffering of a patient with cancer pain (Ref. 31).

Key chapter summary points

- Cancer pain is compounded by understandably associated psychological factors
- Morphine stigma can result in poor compliance and uncontrolled pain
- Shared decision making is essential in cancer pain management
- A trusting patient-clinician partnership is needed
- Clinician's empathy can ease patient's overall suffering

References

3. Melzack R, Wall P D. The challenge of pain 2008. Penguin Books Limited.
31. Greer S, Joseph M. Palliative Care: A Holistic Discipline. *Integrative cancer therapies* 2015; 1-5.

Chapter 7

NON-PHARMACOLOGICAL APPROACH TO CANCER PAIN MANAGEMENT

Recognition

It is important to recognise pharmacological dose ceiling in order to protect medication safety. In this regard, clinical judgement should take precedence over undue reliance on dosage guidelines (Ref. 17).

The clinician may need to consider additional non-pharmacological therapies in cancer pain management. When pain control proves challenging, these measures can be complementary.

Coeliac plexus block

In resistant retroperitoneal pain from pancreatic cancer, neural blockade of the coeliac nerve plexus can augment pharmacological management (Ref. 19).

Trans-cutaneous electrical nerve stimulation (TENS)

This treatment uses the putative *gate control theory* in the spinal dorsal horn. The electrical vibration is conducted by the fast acting, thick walled, heavily myelinated A-Beta nerve fibres which reach the spinal dorsal horn sooner than the pain conducting A-Delta or the C-fibres and block them (Ref. 19).

Relaxation

This is known to reduce the *dis-inhibition* and enhance the descending pain inhibitory pathways (Ref. 3).

Art therapy

The principle of this therapy is based on the patient releasing emotions via art or painting. It can unleash hidden emotional distress which can contribute to difficult pain management in cancer.

Cognitive behavioural therapy (CBT)

Some patients with cancer are unable to focus on their life as the memory of *cancer* is overpowering. This can contribute to difficulty in pain management. CBT helps to reward each positive step made by the patient. Over a course of six weeks of this therapy, the patient is often able to minimise the distress from the memory of *cancer* and focus on living life as best as possible (Ref. 27, 28, 29, 31).

Key chapter summary points

- Recognition of pharmacological ceiling in order to protect medication safety is crucial
- The complexity of cancer pain can require additional non-pharmacological management
- Interventional pain management can complement pharmacological management
- The principle of *gate control theory* has its usefulness in the mechanism of TENS

- Psychological adjunctive therapy proves useful in complex *cancer* pain management

References

3. Melzack R, Wall P D. The challenge of pain 2008. Penguin Books Limited.

17. Wilcock A, Howard P, Charlesworth S. *Palliative care formulary 7.* Pharmaceutical Press, 2020.

19. Bennett M. Neuropathic pain. Oxford university press, 2006.

27. Watson M, Havilland J S, Greer S, Davidson J, Bliss J M. Influence of psychological response on survival in breast cancer: a population-based cohort study, *Lancet* 1999, 354: 1331-1336.

28. Kuchler T, Bestmann B, Rapport S. Impact of psychotherapeutic support for patients with gastrointestinal *cancer* undergoing surgery: 10-year survival results of a randomised trial. *J Clin Oncol.* 2007;25: 2702-2708.

29. Anderson B L, Yang M C, Farrar W B, *et al.* Psychological intervention improves survival

for breast cancer patients. *Cancer*. 2008; 113: 3450-3458.
31. Greer S, Joseph M. Palliative Care: A Holistic Discipline. *Integrative cancer therapies* 2015; 1-5.

Chapter 8

MANAGING CANCER PAIN IN THE DYING PATIENT

Absolute clinical expertise with empathy is required in managing cancer pain in the dying stage. Inability to verbalise when pain is rapidly worsening, heightened by emotional distress compounds the situation. Impaired oral intake and diminishing renal function impact on mode and type of pain management. Family distress needs to be addressed with compassion and understanding.

Rapidly worsening pain

Cancer progression infiltrating visceral organs and nerve sheaths made worse by possible tumour bleeds from fragile blood vessels is the likely cause of rapidly worsening pain in the dying patient.

Inability to verbalise

Extreme exhaustion and inevitable degree of sedation in the dying stage for comfort can impact on the patient's ability to vocalise pain. Body language and facial expressions become crucial in pain assessment. A caring, gentle and sympathetic voice is essential as hearing is known to be intact until the very end of life.

Inability to use oral route

Pain control at this stage needs to be via a continuous sub-cutaneous infusion (CSCI) which is also commonly referred to as a syringe driver, since the patient will not be able to swallow safely. Miscibility of medications through the CSCI should be taken into account. It is recommended that no more than 3 medications are used together in order to optimise absorption.

Type of opioid

If renal function is known to be satisfactory, morphine is used. If the estimated glomerular filtration rate, known as the e-GFR, is reduced between 15 ml per minute and 30 ml per minute, oxycodone is safer. In significant renal impairment with an e-GFR less than 15 ml per minute, alfentanil is advised provided its use is familiar. Otherwise, a small dose oxycodone is considered safe and effective.

Morphine 10mg or oxycodone 5mg or alfentanil 500micrograms can be started and administered over 24 hours in a CSCI and increased according to the patient's need for adequate analgesia.

The CSCI can be in combination with an existing trans-dermal opioid.

If however, the patient was previously receiving an oral opioid, then this dose is converted to 50% in the CSCI and increased according to the patient's analgesic need in order to provide maximum comfort in the dying stage.

Miscibility of medications in a CSCI

In addition to analgesia, additional medications may be required to control agitation or vomiting. The benzodiazepine, midazolam is useful as an anxiolytic agent as it can additionally provide amnesia for painful memories. The phenothiazine, Levomepromazine can provide antiemetic, analgesic and tranquilising effects in the dying patient (Ref. 17). Anti-muscarinic drug, glycopyrronium bromide can provide useful anti-secretory effect in reducing excess respiratory tract secretions in the dying stage.

Supporting the family

Sensitive and empathetic communication is important particularly when the patient is dying. Fear of the patient dying in pain and distress is understandable. In addition to explanation regarding attempts with pain control and providing tranquillity, empathy should be used in understanding their inevitable distress of losing a 'loved one' (Ref. 32).

Key chapter summary points

- Cancer pain can rapidly worsen in the dying stage
- Inability to verbalise or swallow requires extra care in assessment and management
- A continuous sub-cutaneous infusion is used for analgesia and comfort

- Families require understanding, compassion and empathy in the patient's dying stage

References

17. Wilcock A, Howard P, Charlesworth S. *Palliative care formulary 7.* Pharmaceutical Press 2020.
32. NICE guidance. Care in the last days of life: 2015

REFERENCES

1. International association for the study of pain- IASP
2. Saarto T. Palliative care and oncology: the case for early integration. *Eur J Palliative Care.* 2014; 21:109
3. Melzack. R, Wall P D. The challenge of pain 2008. Penguin Books Limited
4. Lynch M E, Craig K D, Peng P W H. Clinical pain management: a practical guide: 2011 Blackwell Publishing Limited
5. Hoskin and Makin. Oncology for Palliative Medicine: 1998 Oxford medical publications
6. Souhami and Tobias. Cancer and its management: 1987 Blackwell Scientific Publications
7. Davis M, Walsh D. cancer pain syndromes. *Euro. J. Pall. Care.* 2000; 7(6)

8. Leon-Casasola O A D. cancer pain: 2006; *Saunders Elsevier (www.elsevier.com)*

9. Mao J. Opioid induced abnormal pain sensitivity: Implications in clinical opioid therapy. Pain 2002. 100: 213-7

10. Mercadante S, Arcuri E. Hyperalgesia and opioid switching. *Am J Hospice Palliative Care* 2005. 22: 291-4

11. Angst M S, Clark J D. Opioid induced hyperalgesia: a qualitative systematic review. Anaesthesiology 2006. 104: 570-87

12. Fallon M. Opioid induced hyperalgesia: fact or fiction? : *Palliative Medicine* 2008. 22: 5-6

13. Bannister K. Opioid induced hyperalgesia-lost in translation? The 10th Annual Royal Marsden pain and opioid conference 2017

14. Virani F. Opioid induced hyperalgesia. *BMJ specialist palliative care* 2020

15. Bennett M. palliative medication: drugs for neuropathic pain. *Euro .J. Pall. Care 2010*; 17(4)

16. Dickenson A. The science of opioids. The 10th Annual Royal Marsden pain and opioid conference 2017
17. Wilcock A, Howard P, Charlesworth S. *Palliative care formulary 7.* Pharmaceutical Press, 2020
18. Smith H. Drugs for pain 2002: ISBN 1-56053-511-3
19. Bennett M. Neuropathic pain. Oxford university press, 2006
20. Rayment *et al.* Neuropathic cancer pain: prevalence, severity, analgesia and impact from European palliative care research collaborative: *Palliative Medicine* 2013. 8: 27
21. Theobald D E, Kirsh K L, Holtsclan E *et al.* An open-label cross-over trial of mirtazapine (15mg & 30mg) in *cancer* patients with pain and other distressing symptoms. *J. Pain Symptom Management*. 2002. 23: 442-447
22. Montgomery S A. Safety of mirtazapine: a review. *Int.clin.psych.pharm.*1995. 10:4,37-45

23. Boer T D. the pharmacologic profile of mirtazapine: *J. Clin. Psychiatry 1996;* 57 (suppl.4)
24. Prommer E. Ketamine for pain: an update for uses in palliative care. *J. palliative. med.* 2012. 4:474-83
25. Mercadante S. opioid combination: rationale and possible clinical applications: *Annals of palliative medicine.* 2013; Vol 2, No 4
26. Reddy A *et al.* Dual opioid therapy using methadone as a co-analgesic: *Expert Opin. Drug Saf.* 2015; 14 (1); 181-183
27. Watson M, Havilland J S, Greer S, Davidson J, Bliss J M. Influence of psychological response on survival in breast cancer: a population-based cohort study, *Lancet.* 1999; 354: 1331-1336
28. Kuchler T, Bestmann B, Rapport S. Impact of psychotherapeutic support for patients with gastrointestinal cancer undergoing surgery: 10-year survival results of a randomised trial. *J Clin Oncol.* 2007;25: 2702-2708.

29. Anderson B L, Yang M C, Farrar W B, *et al.* Psychological intervention improves survival for breast cancer patients. *Cancer.* 2008; 113: 3450-3458.

30. Joseph M, Tayar R. Spinal cord compression requires early detection. *Eur J Palliative Care.* 2005;12: 141-143.

31. Greer S, Joseph M. Palliative Care: A Holistic Discipline. *Integrative cancer therapies* 2015; 1-5

32. NICE guidance. Care in the last days of life: 2015

33. British National Formulary

www.ingramcontent.com/pod-product-compliance
Lightning Source LLC
Chambersburg PA
CBHW070307120526
44590CB00017B/2583